618
SYM ①
Ⓜ

PRINCE CHARLES HOSPITAL
MERTHYR TYDFIL

PC   D0348979

Color Atlas of

OBSTETRICS AND GYNECOLOGY

Color Atlas of

OBSTETRICS AND GYNECOLOGY

E. Malcolm Symonds MD FRCOG
Foundation Professor of Obstetrics and Gynaecology
University of Nottingham
and
Consultant Obstetrician and Gynaecologist
Queen's Medical Centre
Nottingham

Marion B. A. Macpherson DM MRCOG
Consultant Obstetrician and Gynaecologist
Queen's Medical Centre
Nottingham

Ⅵ Mosby-Wolfe

Copyright © 1994 Times Mirror International Publishers Limited
Published in 1994 by Mosby–Wolfe Publishing, an imprint of Times Mirror International Publishers Limited
Printed by Grafos S. A. Arte sobre papel, Barcelona, Spain.
ISBN 0 7234 15897

All rights reserved. No part of this publication may be reproduced, stored in a retrieval system, copied or transmitted, in any form or by any means, electronic, mechanical, photocopying, recording or otherwise without written permission from the Publisher or in accordance with the provisions of the Copyright Act 1956 (as amended), or under the terms of any licence permitting limited copying issued by the Copyright Licensing Agency, 33–34 Alfred Place, London, WC1E 7DP.

Any person who does any unauthorised act in relation to this publication may be liable to criminal prosecution and civil claims for damages.

Permission to photocopy or reproduce solely for internal or personal use is permitted for libraries or other users registered with the Copyright Clearance Center, 21 Congress Street, Salem, MA 01970. This consent does not extend to other kinds of copying, such as copying for general distribution, for advertising or promotional purposes, for creating new collected works, or for resale.

For full details of all Time Mirror International Publishers Limited titles please write to Times Mirror International Publishers Limited, Lynton House, 7–12 Tavistock Square, London WC1H 9LB, England.

A CIP catalogue record for this book is available from the British Library.

Library of Congress Cataloging-in-Publication Data has been applied for.

CONTENTS

Acknowledgements   vi

Preface   vii

1. Methods of examination   9
Obstetrics   9
  Pelvic examination   13
The gynaecological examination   14
  Pelvic examination   15

2. Fetoplacental growth and development   17
Placenta   19

3. Congenital abnormalities and prenatal diagnosis 23
Prenatal screening   23
Most common congenital abnormalities   23

4. Medical disorders of pregnancy   29

5. Antepartum and intrapartum monitoring   31

6. Spontaneous vaginal delivery and breech delivery 35
Spontaneous vaginal delivery   35
Breech delivery   37
Repair of the episiotomy   41

7. Operative deliveries   43
Caesarean section   43
Epidural anaesthesia   49
Low forceps delivery   50

8. Ultrasound and magnetic resonance imaging   55
Ultrasound imaging   55
  Congenital abnormalities   60
  Gynaecological conditions   62
Magnetic resonance imaging   64
  Fetus and placenta   64
  Gynaecology   65

9. Gynaecology   67
Anatomy of the pelvic organs   67
Histology of the endometrium   72

10. Lesions of the vulva and vagina   75
Congenital abnormailities of the vagina   75
Lesions of the vulva   78
Vulvar disease   80

11. The Cervix   83
Cervical cytology   87

12. Lesions of the uterus and fallopian tubes   89
Developmental abnormalities   89
Tumours   90
Endometriosis   93
Lesions of the fallopian tube   94

13. Lesions of the ovary   97
Follicular cyst   97
Endometriosis   98
Benign cysts   100
Malignant tumours of the ovary   101

14. Common gynaecological operations   105
Abdominal hysterectomy   105
Vaginal hysterectomy   108
Dilatation of the cervix and endometrial curettage   112
Laparascopy   113
Open clip sterilisation   115
Minimal invasive surgery   116
Laparascopic oophorectomy   118

Index   119

ACKNOWLEDGEMENTS

In this atlas, we have attempted to collect together all the slides and photographs needed to give an overview of the common conditions observed in obstetrics and gynaecology. The majority of the photographs have been produced at the Queen's Medical Centre, Nottingham, but some images have been collected from other centres and contributors.

We are greatly indebted to the Audio-Visual Department at the Queen's Medical Centre and in particular Mr Geoffrey Gilbert for their assistance over many years. We are also indebted to Mr Robert Hammond for providing pictures of vulval carcinomas; Mr Tony Hollingworth for his assistance with pictures in the section on cervical pathology; Dr Jane Johnson and Dr Malcolm Anderson for their assistance with pictures of gynaecological pathology, Dr Peter Twining and Mrs Jo Swallow for providing a large number of ultrasound images; Professor Brian Worthington and Mr Martin Powell for the pictures on magnetic resonance imaging; Dr Simon Fishel for providing the embryology pictures, and Dr Norman Thomas who both performed and photographed the anatomical prosections. Dr Derek Johnson provided pictures of some of the congenital anomalies. We are also indebted to Mr Marcus Filshie and Mr Martin Powell for the pictures of minimal invasive surgery.

Finally, we owe a great debt of gratitude to all those patients who so kindly agreed, albeit anonymously, to appear in print. Although care has been taken to ensure anonymity, the authors apologise for any oversight in this regard.

We hope that readers of this atlas get some information from the wide range of pictures and pathologies. Although the atlas contains over 400 pictures, it is by no means comprehensive. Like all such works, it bears the hallmark of the authors' preferences, but we hope it will provide a firm pictorial basis for obstetrics and gynaecology in both undergraduate and postgraduate studies.

Marion B.A. Macpherson, DM, MRCOG
E. Malcolm Symonds, MD, FRCOG

PREFACE

Obstetrics and gynaecology are generally visual subjects. They lend themselves well to illustrative material. Indeed, gynaecological pathology often has a spectacular dimension and the appearances of any tumour lend themselves well to the visual memory.

We compiled this atlas as a combined photographic record, bearing in mind that many students have limited time in which to study this subject in medical school. The atlas is also presented as an aid to practising clinicians to remind them of common conditions of pregnancy and of gynaecological pathology. The collection is by no means comprehensive. It must be taken as complementary to other presentations which limit the subject to one specialised topic.

Some of the photographs in this atlas have been collected over the last 20 years, but the majority of the obstetric presentations have been collected within the last two years and are new, previously unpublished material.

Nothing can suitably illustrate obstetric procedures in a static form, but these images, if considered in conjunction with line drawings, provide a useful reminder and illustration of common obstetric procedures.

The ovaries, because of their totipotential nature, produce a wide variety of benign and malignant tumours. No attempt has been made to amass a comprehensive collection. Furthermore, many tumours have an appearance that can only be diagnosed histologically and it has not been our intention to present this book as an atlas of histology.

Some surgical techniques have been included to illustrate the pathology or structural abnormalities of the genital tract better and provide photographic material of common procedures that can be used to educate both practitioners and patients.

Marion B.A. Macpherson, DM, MRCOG
E. Malcolm Symonds, MD, FRCOG

PRINCE CHARLES HOSPITAL
MERTHYR TYDFIL

1. Methods of examination

Obstetrics

Pregnancy produces changes in every system in the body in the process of achieving preparation for parturition and the support of the newborn child. Some of these changes are obvious and readily apparent and others are of a more subtle nature and are less specific.

At the initial visit to clinic, a complete physical examination is performed. Height is recorded and the weight is recorded at the first and all subsequent visits. Blood pressure is recorded with the patient supine and in the lateral supine position to avoid vena caval compression (**1.1**). Diastolic blood pressure is usually taken as the Korotkoff fourth sound, although there has been some recent shift to recording values that relate to the disappearance of the sound.

Skin pigmentation (**1.2**) is most noticeable on the forehead and the cheeks, particularly in women of darker complexion and from sunny climates.

1.1 Blood pressure is recorded from the right arm. Cuff size is important. Posture should be consistent and blood pressure is usually taken with the mother lying supine with a left lateral tilt to relieve any pressure of the enlarged pregnant uterus from the inferior vena cava. The diastolic blood pressure in pregnancy is recorded as the fourth Korotkoff sound.

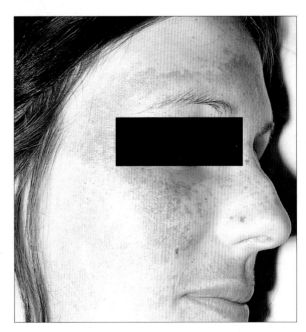

1.2 Chloasma—the 'mask of pregnancy'. Pigmentation occurs across the forehead and the cheeks in some women during pregnancy and later disappears.

Breast changes include an increase in size and vascularity as well as increased areolar pigmentation and the development of Montgomery's tubercles (**1.3–1.5**).

1.3 Breast changes in pregnancy. These include enlargement, increased vascularity, and the production of colostrum.

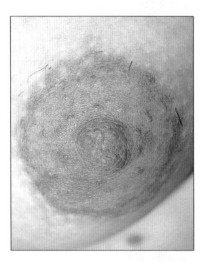

1.4 The areola of the nipple. This shows increased pigmentation and the development of raised sebaceous glands known as Montgomery's tubercles.

1.5 The areola. This shows marked pigmentation in women with dark skins.

Striae gravidarum do not become apparent on the abdomen, thighs and breasts of all pregnant women, but may be particularly florid in some women, leaving silvery abdominal scars after the pregnancy (**1.6–1.7**).

1.6 Lateral inspection of the abdomen in advanced pregnancy. This shows the presence of striae gravidarum, which extend onto the breasts and the lateral surface of the thighs and buttocks.

1.7 Direct view of the anterior abdominal wall in the third trimester of pregnancy. The scars are initially purplish in colour and appear in lines of stress in the skin. In subsequent pregnancies, the scars are silvery white in appearance.

Abdominal examination is particularly important in assessing fetal growth and development. Serial measurements of fundal height allow a reasonable measurement of fetal growth (**1.8–1.10**).

1.8 Palpation of the uterine fundus at 18 weeks' gestation. The border of the hand is placed along the superior margin of the uterine fundus.

1.9 By 36 weeks' gestation. The uterine fundus lies in apposition to the xiphisternum.

1.10 Measurement of the fundal height allows assessment of gestational age and fetal size. Serial measurements are particularly useful in the assessment of fetal growth.

Palpation of the fetal parts enables determination of fetal lie, presentation and attitude, as well as the station of the presenting part (**1.11–1.14**).

1.11 Palpation of the presenting part and the position of the back. These are important routine observations.

1.12 Pawlik's grip. This enables the attendant to assess the degree of descent of the presenting part. It should be used with gentleness because, if applied roughly, it may be uncomfortable for the mother.

1.13 Checking for the presence of excessive amniotic fluid or hydramnios. This involves eliciting the presence of a fluid thrill. A hand placed centrally dampens down vibrations in the subcutaneous fat.

1.14 Auscultation of the fetal heart. The Pinard stethoscope is applied firmly at right angles to the abdominal wall. The instrument should not be held in the hand during auscultation because this may muffle the sound.

Pelvic examination

At the first visit, a pelvic examination is performed to exclude any pathology and to assess the size and position of the uterus. Pregnancy induces marked changes in the vaginal walls with increased vascularity and transudation (**1.15**). The cervix also undergoes enlargement, softening and increased vascularity.

1.15 Speculum examination. This reveals the increased vascularity and engorgement of the vaginal walls in pregnancy.

Assessment of the bony pelvis involves palpation for the sacral promontory (**1.16**), observation of the sacral curve (**1.17**), and identification of the ischial spines (**1.18**), the angle of the subpubic arch (**1.19**), and the intertuberous diameter. Urine analysis is performed at each antenatal visit and tested for protein, glucose and ketone bodies.

1.16 Assessment of the bony pelvis. Feeling for the sacral promontory allows an assessment of the anteroposterior diameter of the pelvic inlet.

1.17 Palpation of the sacral curve and the attitude of the coccyx. This is important in the assessment of the pelvic cavity.

1.18 The ischial spines represent the lateral limits of the narrowest plane in the pelvis. The top of the finger can be seen in apposition to the right ischial spine.

1.19 The normal subpubic angle is 90°. A narrow subpubic angle indicates both a narrow pelvic outlet and often a funnel pelvis.

The gynaecological examination

The approach to any clinical problem in any discipline in medicine involves obtaining a detailed medical and surgical history as well as a detailed history of the presenting complaint. Examination of a patient presenting with gynaecological symptoms also involves a general examination with particular assessment of the breasts (**1.20–1.23**) and abdomen (**1.24**).

1.20 Inspection of the breasts. This should be a routine part of the gynaecological examination.

1.21 The breast should be systematically inspected. The position and mobility of any breast lumps can then be defined.

1.22 Palpation of the inner quadrants of the breast. This should form part of a systematic routine.

1.23 Palpation of the axillary tail. This is particularly important as assessment must include all breast tissue.

1.24 Examination of the abdomen may show distension. A view from a lateral aspect, as in this case, shows the outline of a large ovarian cyst with central dullness to percussion.

Pelvic examination

Pelvic examination (**1.25–1.31**) involves speculum inspection and bimanual examination. Both procedures are equally important.

- **A cervical smear** is taken where appropriate after inspecting the cervix (see **1.27–1.29**).

- **Bimanual examination** (see **1.30**) is used to assess the size, shape, and position of the uterus, and the presence of any adnexal tumours.

  The essence of good pelvic examination is to obtain the maximum information with minimal discomfort.

1.25 Inspection of the vulva. Pelvic examination involves inspection of the vulva. Look for vulval lesions and note the general condition of the vulval skin.

1.26 Inspection of the vaginal walls. Insertion of a bivalve or Cuscoe's speculum allows inspection of the vaginal walls.

1.27 Inspection of the cervix. Insertion of a bivalve or Cuscoe's speculum also allows inspection of the cervix.

1.28 Cervical smear. A cervical smear is taken with an Ayre's speculum.

1.29 Cervical smear. The material obtained by scraping the cervix is placed on a glass slide for fixation and staining.

1.30 Bimanual palpation of the pelvic organs. The pelvic examination is completed by bimanual palpation of the pelvic organs. Palpation of the fornices is important to detect adrenal masses.

1.31 Colposcopy. Sometimes a more detailed examination of the cervix is indicated. A colposcope allows a close inspection of cervical epithelium.

2. Fetoplacental growth and development

Fertilisation occurs when spermatozoa reach the oocyte (**2.1–2.6**) in the ampulla of the tube. After the nucleus of the sperm head passes into the cytoplasm of the oocyte, the second polar body of the oocyte is expelled.

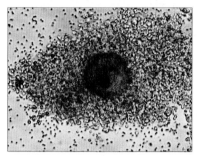

2.1 The oocyte/cumulus complex. At the moment of aspiration from a human Graafian follicle.

2.2 An unfertilised egg in metaphase II.

2.3 A bi-ovular zona pellucida or a fused zona pellucida containing two oocytes. One oocyte appears to be mature, but the other contains a germinal vesicle and is slightly degenerate.

2.4 Subzonal insemination. The injection of spermatozoa into the perivitelline space is facilitated by slightly dehydrating the oocyte. Microinjection is performed with a needle 11 microns in diameter and a holding pipette about 30 microns in diameter.

2.5 Micro-injection. High magnification view.

2.6 A one-cell egg with sperm in the perivitelline space.

As the conceptus passes down the tube, it undergoes cleavage (**2.7–2.9**) and, at the 16-cell stage, forms the morula and then the blastocyst (**2.10–2.12**). Implantation occurs six days after ovulation. Subsequent development of the fetus occurs initially as the result of a massive increase in the number of cells in the inner cell mass, but with relatively little increase in the mass.

2.7 A two-cell pronucleate human oocyte. 18 hours after insemination *in vitro.*

2.8 A three-cell pronucleate human oocyte with several attendants on the surface of the zona pellucida.

2.9 A six-cell human embryo. 49 hours after insemination *in vitro.*

2.10 Early human morula. 74 hours post insemination *in vitro.*

2.11 A late human morula and blastocyst. Note the small cavitation and presence of blastocoelic fluid in the late morula and the full blastocoelic cavity and inner cell mass.

2.12 Blastocyst. High-power view at 5.5 days post insemination.

The major processes of organogenesis are complete by 12 weeks' gestation (**2.13**), but the development of function in the various systems continues at different rates. There is a heartbeat by five weeks' gestation and fetal respiration is established *in utero* by 12 weeks. Mucosal glands appear in the gut by 16 weeks (**2.14 and 2.15**) and by 26 weeks most of the digestive enzymes are present. Functional development of the fetal kidney favours early development of the renal tubules before glomerular function occurs and fetal urine makes a significant contribution to amniotic fluid.

2.13 At 12 weeks' gestation. The fetus reacts to stimuli. The upper limbs reach their final relative length and the fetal sex is distinguishable externally.

2.14 At 16 weeks' gestation. Crown–rump length is 122 mm. Lower limbs achieve their final relative length and the eyes face anteriorly.

2.15 At 24 weeks' gestation. The fetal lungs have started to secrete surfactant.

Placenta

The placenta has a vital function in gaseous exchange, fetal nutrition, and the manipulation of maternal physiology to the advantage of the fetus. The functional unit of the placenta is the stem villus. These develop from the chorion frondosum and the remaining 'non-placental' portion of the chorion frondosum eventually forms the chorion laeve as part of the fetal membranes (**2.16**). The amnion lies inside the chorion and is loosely attached to it (**2.17**).

2.16 The fetal surface of the placenta. This shows the chorionic plate and the fetal vessels.

2.17 The fetal membranes. These consist of the two layers of chorion and the amnion.

The maternal surface of the placenta exhibits a series of cotyledons (**2.18–2.21**), which are clusters of fetal villi. At term the mature placenta weighs approximately 600 g. The cotyledon may become infarcted (**2.22**) and if this occurs in sufficient numbers fetal growth is impaired. The umbilical cord contains two arteries and one vein surrounded by Wharton's jelly and amnion. The vessels have a helical disposition.

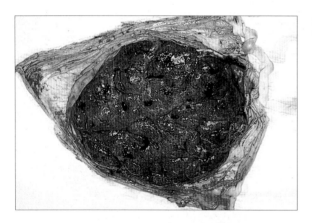

2.18 Maternal surface of the full-term placenta. This shows the cotyledonary structure.

2.19 Fetal surface of a circumvallate placenta. There is reduplication of the membrane at the rim of the placenta.

2.20 Placental abruption. This leaves the maternal surface covered with blood clot.

2.21 A twin placenta with fusion of the two placentae, which appear to be indistinguishable. The two umbilical cords can be seen.

2.22 Placenta showing multiple white infarcted cotyledons. These affect nearly half the placental surface.

3. Congenital abnormalities and prenatal diagnosis

The incidence of major congenital abnormalities varies from country to country. In the UK, the figure has been estimated at 25–30/1000 births.

Prenatal screening

Prenatal screening (**3.1–3.9**) includes:
- Biochemical tests such as alpha fetoprotein, combined alpha fetoprotein, HCG and serum oestriol.
- Chorion villus sampling.
- Amniocentesis
- Ultrasound screening, now the major technique for imaging structural abnormalities.

Most common congenital abnormalities

The five most common groups of congenital abnormalities (**3.10–3.24**) include:
- Neural tube defects.
- Congenital heart disease.
- Severe mental retardation.
- Down's syndrome.
- Hare lip/cleft palate.

3.2 Chorion villus sampling. Chorion villus sampling needle.

3.1 Chorion villus sampling. Schematic representation of chorion villus biopsy. A small sample of chorionic tissue is taken either vaginally through the cervix or via the abdominal route.

3.3 Amniocentesis. Preparation of the maternal anterior abdominal wall for amniocentesis.

3.4 Amniocentesis. Infiltration of local anaesthetic over the placement site of the amniocentesis needle.

3.5 Amniocentesis. Insertion of the amniocentesis needle into a pool of amniotic fluid detected by ultrasound.

3.6 Amniocentesis. Aspiration of amniotic fluid with a 20 ml syringe.

3.7 Amniocentesis. Alliquoting of the amniotic fluid for cell culture and biochemistry.

3.9 Fetoscopy. Needle endoscope used for fetoscopy.

3.8 Fetoscopy. Direct visualisation of the fetus through an endoscope is now rarely used.

3.10 Anencephaly. The cerebral hemisphere and cranial vault are absent.

3.11 Lumbar myelomeningocoele. The defect in the posterior bony aspect of the vertebrae exposes the spinal membranes.

3.12 Meningomyelocoele of the cervical spine. A similar defect high in the spinal canal.

3.13 Small open neural tube defect. This was identified by high amniotic fluid alpha fetoprotein levels and confirmed at the time of abortion.

3.14 Gross exomphalus. Shortly after delivery of a mature infant by Caesarean section.

3.15 Gross exomphalus: successful closure of the abdominal wall defect. This was performed immediately after delivery.

3.16 Large encephalocoele. Lateral view.

3.17 Large encephalocoele. Posterior view.

3.18 Large cystic hygroma. This was detected by ultrasound scan.

3.19 Grossly hydropic fetus associated with trisomy.

3.20 Potter's syndrome. This syndrome is associated with renal agenesis and is incompatible with life when there is complete renal agenesis. The 'crumpled ears' reflect poor cartilage development and the effects of severe oligohydramnios.

3.21 Down's syndrome. Facial appearance of an infant with Down's syndrome. (Courtesy of Dr. D.I. Johnston.)

3.22 Turner's syndrome. This syndrome is associated with pedal and lower limb oedema and chromosome analysis of 45XO.

3.23 Caudal regimen syndrome (sacral agenesis) in an infant of a diabetic mother. (Courtesy of Dr. D.I. Johnston.)

3.24 Congenital adrenal hyperplasia (21-hydroxylase deficiency). This female infant shows clitoromegaly and labioscrotal fusion. (Courtesy of Dr. D.I. Johnston.)

4. Medical disorders of pregnancy

The majority of medical complications encountered in pregnancy do not present with physical signs. However, some common conditions are shown in this brief section (**4.1–4.10**). Most of the medical conditions do not exhibit any specific visual signs and cannot therefore be represented macroscopically by visual images.

4.1 Subconjunctival ecchymosis following normal delivery. The rupture of subconjunctival vessels follows the straining that occurs in the second stage of labour.

4.2 Macroscopic features of an infant born to a mother with insulin-dependent diabetes. The child has increased subcutaneous fat and generalised visceromegaly.

4.3 Facial oedema and severe pre-eclampsia. Oedema commonly occurs in the limb extremities, over the face, and the abdominal wall.

4.4 Facial oedema and severe pre-eclampsia. Lateral view.

4.5 Thyroid enlargement in a normal pregnancy. Some degree of goitre is physiologically normal.

4.6 Thyroid enlargement. Close up view.

4.7 Thyroid enlargement. In profile. It is often difficult to differentiate between normal and abnormal thyroid enlargement in pregnancy.

4.8 Herpes gestationis on the abdomen. This is a rare condition that arises only during pregnancy and disappears after delivery.

4.9 Herpes gestationis on the abdomen. Lateral view.

4.10 Herpes gestationis on the thigh.

5. Antepartum and intrapartum monitoring

Antepartum and intrapartum monitoring are standard techniques of fetal assessment.

- Antenatally, the fetal heart rate is monitored by pulsed Doppler ultrasound (**5.1–5.5**).
- During the course of labour, fetal heart rate can be monitored directly by applying an electrode to the fetal presenting part using the fetal ECG. The heart rate and uterine activity are recorded and the heart rate is displayed in an analogue tracing so that patterns of heart rate change can be identified (**5.6–5.13**). More recently, techniques have been developed to show the features of the fetal ECG waveform in real time displays.

These techniques have been developed in an attempt to detect fetal asphyxia. Fetal acid–base balance can be measured directly in labour by sampling scalp blood taken from the presenting parts (**5.14–5.16**).

The baseline heart rate is the number of beats per minute between alterations, and lies between 120 to 160 beats/minute. Fetal heart rate (FHR) variability is defined as the amplitude of oscillations of the baseline, and where it is greater than 5 beats/ minute, it is considered to be normal. An amplitude of between 3–5 beats/minute is often associated with sleep patterns, and is only significant if associated with other FHR abnormalities. A flat baseline with a variability of 0–2 beats/minute, when associated with other abnormalities, is considered ominous.

Alterations in the FHR lasting less than 10 minutes include accelerations which are indications of good fetal prognosis and decelerations which may be early, late or variable. The definition is based on the time relationship to uterine contractions. The lag time is defined as the interval between the peak of the contractions and the nadir of the decelerations. In an early deceleration, the lag time is less than 18 seconds; in the late deceleration it is greater than 18 seconds. Some examples of antenatal CTGs are demonstrated (**5.3–5.5**), and Figures **5.8–5.12** show examples of intrapartum recordings.

5.1 Standard antenatal cardiotocography (CTG). The transducers are applied to the maternal abdomen to detect the fetal heart beat and uterine contractions.

5.2 Standard antenatal CTG. The application of the heart rate transducer attached to the maternal abdominal wall. The mother clasps the event marker in her right hand and presses the button when she feels a fetal movement.

5.3 Normal antenatal CTG. This shows baseline variability of greater than 5 beats/minute.

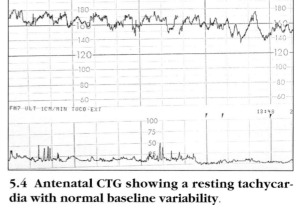

5.4 Antenatal CTG showing a resting tachycardia with normal baseline variability.

5.5 Antenatal CTG with a normal baseline heart rate, but no baseline variability.

5.6 Copeland electrode. The Copeland electrode is used for direct application to the fetal presenting part in labour.

5.7 Copeland electrode. Single coil of the Copeland disposable electrode.

5.8 Normal intrapartum recording. This shows a normal baseline heart rate and normal baseline variability. The uterine contractions can be seen on the bottom line.

5.9 Baseline bradycardia with loss of heart rate variability during the first stage of labour.

5.10 Early decelerations. The peak of the deceleration coinciding with the zenith of the uterine contraction.

5.11 Profound and persistent bradycardia with slow recovery to a normal heart rate.

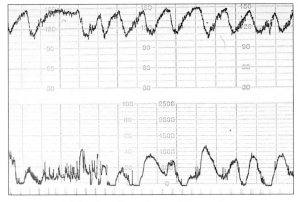

5.12 Variable decelerations. These do not appear to be related to the uterine contractions.

5.13 Complications of a fetal scalp electrode. This shows two ulcerated areas associated with hair loss.

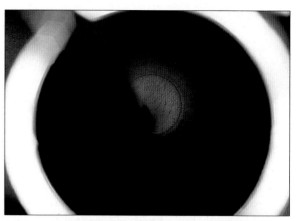

5.14 Sampling fetal scalp blood: the amnioscope. This is introduced through the cervical os to display the fetal presenting part. It consists of an obturator and a cannula.

5.15 Sampling fetal scalp blood. A sharp blade is introduced on a long holder to incise the scalp.

5.16 Sampling fetal scalp blood. A drop of blood can be seen to form on the fetal scalp and can then be aspirated into a fetal capillary and submitted for fetal acid–base balance measurement.

6. Spontaneous vaginal delivery and breech delivery

Spontaneous vaginal delivery

Normal spontaneous vaginal delivery (**6.1–6.9**) is associated with progressive flexion and descent of the head, distension of the pelvic floor, delivery of the head, restitution and external rotation and delivery of the shoulders and trunk. Placental delivery is achieved by cord traction and fundal pressure.

6.1 Spontaneous vaginal delivery: the second stage of labour. The scalp becomes visible with contractions and expulsive efforts by the mother.

6.2 Spontaneous vaginal delivery: crowning of the head. The perineum is distended until the head crowns.

6.3 Spontaneous vaginal delivery: at delivery. The head is in the anteroposterior position at delivery.

6.4 Spontaneous vaginal delivery: delivery of the head and shoulders. Delivery of the head is accompanied by external rotation so that the occiput rotates from the anterior position to a point laterally. The anterior shoulder is delivered by downward traction on the head and the posterior shoulder by anterior traction.

PRINCE CHARLES HOSPITAL
MERTHYR TYDFIL

6.5 Spontaneous vaginal delivery: the third stage of labour. The abdomen is palpated to make sure that the uterine fundus is contracted. The placenta appears distending the vulva.

6.6 Spontaneous vaginal delivery: placental delivery. The placenta is delivered with cord traction and counter pressure against the uterine fundus.

6.7 Spontaneous vaginal delivery: after delivery. The cord is clamped and cut and the infant is weighed.

6.8 Spontaneous vaginal delivery: after delivery. The perineum, vulva, and vaginal wall are checked for lacerations.

6.9 Spontaneous vaginal delivery: face presentation. Abnormal facial bruising followed spontaneous vaginal delivery as a face presentation.

Breech delivery

In a breech presentation (**6.10–6.26**), the buttocks are expelled to the waist, the limbs are lifted out by flexion of the thighs and knees and the trunk is allowed to hang until the head enters the pelvis. Delivery of the head is achieved by anterior rotation of the trunk and the application of forceps to the aftercoming head.

6.10 Breech delivery: breech presentation. The anterior buttock appears at the introitus.

6.11 Breech delivery: breech presentation. The vulva and anus are distended by the breech.

6.12 Breech delivery: episiotomy. A mediolateral episiotomy is cut to facilitate descent of the breech and subsequent delivery of the fetal head.

6.13 Breech delivery: episiotomy. Care is taken not to injure the presenting part.

PRINCE CHARLES HOSPITAL
MERTHYR TYDFIL

6.14 Breech delivery: fetal descent. Further descent of the anterior buttock occurs.

6.15 Breech delivery: fetal descent. Both buttocks come into view as well as the anterior thigh.

6.16 Breech delivery: fetal descent. The fetal anus and vulva are now apparent.

6.17 Breech delivery: delivery of the buttocks. The buttocks are expelled by voluntary maternal effort.

6.18 Breech delivery: sacral rotation. The fetal sacrum rotates anteriorly.

6.19 Breech delivery: delivery of the legs. The legs are delivered by flexion of the thighs and knees.

6.20 Breech delivery: delivery of the anterior shoulder.

6.21 Breech delivery: delivery of the posterior shoulder.

6.22 Breech delivery: descent of the head. The trunk is allowed to hang to encourage descent of the head.

6.23 Breech delivery: insertion of the first forceps blade. The trunk of the baby is swung anteriorly and the first forceps blade is inserted.

6.24 Breech delivery: insertion of the second forceps blade. The second blade is applied and locked into position.

6.25 Breech delivery: delivery of the head. Gentle traction is applied to complete a controlled delivery of the head.

6.26 Breech delivery: the third stage of labour.
The third stage is completed by cord traction.

Repair of the episiotomy

Repair of the episiotomy (**6.27–6.32**) is achieved by closure of the vaginal wall, interrupted sutures into the levatores ani, and interrupted sutures to the skin.

6.27 (left) Inspection of the episiotomy. The extent of the wound is assessed.

6.28 (right) Closure of the episiotomy. Care is taken to expose the apex of the incision in the vaginal wall and a continuous absorbable suture is used to close the vaginal wall.

6.29 Closure of the episiotomy. The wound is closed to the introitus.

6.30 Closure of the episiotomy. Care is taken to ensure that the introitus is not constricted.

6.31 Closure of the episiotomy. Interrupted absorbable sutures are inserted into the levatores ani.

6.32 Closure of the episiotomy. Interrupted mattress sutures are used to close the skin.

7. Operative deliveries

Caesarean section

Caesarean section is the most widely used form of operative delivery. The incidence of operative delivery varies considerably between various countries with an incidence of 12 % in the UK and figures in excess of 20 % in the USA. The common indications include:

- Fetal distress.
- Cephalopelvic disproportion.
- Placenta praevia.
- Severe pre-eclampsia.

The increased incidence of Caesarean section is partly related to the desire to reduce fetal loss and partly to the greater safety of the procedure under modern conditions (**7.1–7.24**).

Until the 1940s the common procedure was an upper segment Caesarean section, but this operation was largely abandoned because of the increased risk of uterine scar rupture during the third trimester of pregnancy. Furthermore, the postoperative complications are worse because of the increased risk of paralytic ileus, wound infection, and postpartum haemorrhage.

7.1 Caesarean section: incision. Delivery is effected through a low transverse abdominal incision.

7.2 Caesarean section: incision. The rectus sheath is incised.

7.3 Caesarean section: incision. The rectus sheath is then dissected and cut free of the rectus muscle.

7.4 Caesarean section: incision. The parietal peritoneum is incised and the abdominal cavity is opened.

7.5 Caesarean section: incision. The lower uterine segment is exposed.

7.6 Caesarean section: incision. The peritoneum over the lower segment is incised.

7.7 Caesarean section: incision. The peritoneum is reflected from the lower segment.

7.8 Caesarean section: incision. The uterus is incised transversely and the membranes are exposed.

7.9 Caesarean section: delivery. The amniotic fluid can be seen gushing from the amniotic sac.

7.10 Caesarean section: delivery. A hand is inserted into the uterus to lift out the presenting part.

7.11 Caesarean section: delivery. The presenting par—in this case the breech—is delivered by gentle traction.

7.12 Caesarean section: delivery. The legs are released and the rest of the trunk is delivered to the shoulders.

7.13 Caesarean section: delivery. The shoulders are released by applying torsion to the trunk.

7.14 Caesarean section: delivery. Delivery is completed by applying forceps to the head.

7.15 Caesarean section: delivery. The head is released with gentle traction.

7.16 Caesarean section: placental delivery. The infant is laid on the maternal abdomen, the cord is clamped, and the placenta expelled.

7.17 Caesarean section: placental delivery. The placenta is expelled through the abdominal wound.

7.18 Caesarean section: placental delivery. The uterine cavity is explored to ensure that no placental tissue or fetal membranes are left behind.

7.19 Caesarean section: closure. The edges of the uterine incision are grasped with haemostatic clamps.

7.20 Caesarean section: closure. The first layer of myometrium is closed with a continuous suture.

7.21 Caesarean section: closure. The second and outer layer is sutured.

7.22 Caesarean section: closure. Closure of visceral peritoneum.

7.23 (left) Caesarean section: closure. Closure of the rectus sheath.

7.24 (right) Caesarean section: closure. Closure of the skin wound.

Epidural anaesthesia

Lumbar epidural anaesthesia (**7.25–7.29**) is one of the most widely used methods of pain relief in labour. It is now commonly used as a method of regional anaesthesia for Caesarean section.

7.25 Epidural anaesthesia. The patient is placed on her left side with her thighs and trunk flexed. The position of the spines of the lumbar vertebrae are marked.

7.26 Epidural anaesthesia. The epidural needle is inserted between the vertebral spines of L$_3$ and L$_4$ after infiltration of the skin with local anaesthesia.

7.27 Epidural anaesthesia. The resistance to the injection of a small amount of air is felt to make sure that the tip of the needle is in the epidural space.

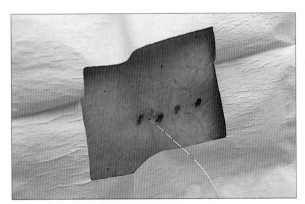

7.28 Epidural anaesthesia. The epidural catheter is inserted through the needle and the needle is then removed.

7.29 Epidural anaesthesia. Epidural 'top ups' are performed by injecting local anaesthesia through a self-sealing valve.

Low forceps delivery

7.30 Low forceps delivery: insertion of the left blade. The left blade of the forceps is inserted and directly applied alongside the head.

7.31 Low forceps delivery: application of the right blade. The right blade of the forceps is now applied to the right side of the pelvis until it lies easily alongside the fetal head.

7.32 Low forceps delivery: locking the blades. The blades are now locked together.

7.33 Low forceps delivery: episiotomy. With the perineum stretched, a mediolateral episiotomy is cut.

7.34 Low forceps delivery: descent. Traction is applied downwards and backwards to release the occiput under the pubic arch.

7.35 Low forceps delivery: descent. Further intermittent traction is applied.

7.36 Low forceps delivery: descent. The scalp can now be clearly seen through the distended vulva.

7.37 Low forceps delivery: crowning of the head. The head is now beginning to crown.

7.38 Low forceps delivery: crowning of the head. Maximum distension of the vulva and perineum occurs.

7.39 Low forceps delivery: delivery. As the head is delivered, the forceps blades are removed.

7.40 Low forceps delivery: delivery. The umbilical cord is around the neck and is loosened before the shoulders are delivered.

7.41 Low forceps delivery: delivery. The anterior shoulder is delivered by downward traction on the head.

7.42 Low forceps delivery: delivery. The umbilical cord is cut and clamped.

7.43 Low forceps delivery: delivery. Delivery of the child is complete. The placenta is still in the uterus.

7.44 Low forceps delivery: placental delivery. After checking that the uterus is firmly contracted, cord traction is applied with suprapubic pressure on the uterus.

7.45 Low forceps delivery: placental delivery. The placenta descends into the vagina.

7.46 Low forceps delivery: placental delivery. The placenta now lies entirely in the vagina and is about to deliver.

7.47 (left) Low forceps delivery: placental delivery. The placental expulsion is complete and the placenta and membranes are examined.

7.48 (right) Low forceps delivery: repair of episiotomy. The episiotomy is sutured.

PRINCE CHARLES HOSPITAL
MERTHYR TYDFIL

8. Ultrasound and magnetic resonance imaging

The introduction of ultrasound in imaging of the female pelvis and the fetus has revolutionised the management of abnormalities in pregnancy and the diagnosis of gynaecological pathology. The images produced in this section are no more than samples to illustrate the value of these techniques in some areas of clinical practice.

Ultrasound imaging

Ultrasound imaging is based on the direction of sound waves with frequencies between 2–20 megahertz into the tissues of the pelvis and abdominal cavity. The returning echoes from tissue interfaces of differing densities are used to construct images of the target site. Ultrasound is produced by the excitation of the piezo-electric crystal. The transmission phase is short and the 'transmitting' crystal reverts to a receiving phase.

Most modern instruments are real-time scanners and are available in three forms.
ı Linear array.
ı Mechanical array.
ı Phased array.

The quality of images continues to improve. However, ultrasound imaging is always limited to demonstrating physical structure (**8.1–8.37**) and not biochemical composition.

8.1 Crown–rump length. The measurement of crown–rump length is demonstrated in this picture and is the technique used in early pregnancy to assess gestational age.

8.2 Crown–rump length. A crown–rump length of 40 mm is demonstrated in this film in early pregnancy.

8.4 At 14 weeks' gestation. The features of the face can now be seen.

8.3 At 13 weeks' gestation. The whole fetus demonstrated in longitudinal section.

8.5 Facial structure. The details of facial structure can be seen with remarkable clarity.

8.6 At 15 weeks' gestation. A normal fetus.

8.7 Fetal spine. The fetal spine can be screened in sufficient detail to allow recognition of spina bifida and is used as a screening procedure.

8.8 A male fetus identified by the external genitalia. This is not always possible and the identification of the sex of the fetus is therefore not always reliable.

8.9 At 18 weeks' gestation. At this time the structures of all organs are screened.

8.10 Fetal heart. Imaging of the four chambers of the fetal heart.

8.11 (left) Fetal heart. A further four-chamber view of the fetal heart showing the foramen ovale.

8.12 (right) Measurement of head circumference. This allows an assessment of fetal growth and gestational age.

8.13 Measurement of head circumference. If the section is too high, assessment of gestational age can be inaccurate.

8.14 Measurement of biparietal diameter. This was the earliest method of assessing gestational age. The diameter in this picture is 82 mm.

8.15 Cerebral ventricles. Demonstration of the cerebral ventricles in a normal fetus.

8.16 Measurement of abdominal circumference. This is valuable in the assessment of asymmetrical growth retardation.

8.17 (left) Doppler blood velocity measurement. The fetal aorta is visible in this film and is used for Doppler blood velocity measurement.

8.18 (right) Umbilical cord. The structure and position of the umbilical cord are seen and can be used for obtaining blood samples from the fetus.

8.19 (left) Twin pregnancy. The early detection of a twin pregnancy has been particularly useful in the management of multiple pregnancies.

8.20 (right) Amniocentesis. This is commonly performed at 16 weeks' gestation. The needle can be seen on this film.

Congenital abnormalities: ultrasound images

8.21 Anencephaly. The cranial vault is missing.

8.22 Hydrocephalus associated with spina bifida.

8.23 Spina bifida. Transverse section.

8.24 Holoprosencephaly. This condition is associated with a fluid-filled cranial vault, a small skull, disorganised cerebral ventricles, and prominent basal nuclei.

8.25 Fetal ascites with fluid distension of the abdominal cavity.

8.26 (left) Gastroschisis with extrusion of the fetal bowel.

8.27 (right) Exomphalos. This defect in the abdominal wall is more severe and the eviscerated organs include small intestine and liver.

Gynaecological conditions: ultrasound images

8.28 (left) Hydatidiform mole. This shows the mottled snow storm appearance of the molar tissue.

8.29 (right) Missed abortion. The conceptus is small and lies inside a disproportionately large sac. The size of the conceptus is not consistent with the gestational age and a fetal heart beat cannot be detected.

8.30 Retained products of conception. Placental tissue can be seen in the uterine cavity.

8.31 Normal endometrium. The thickness of normal endometrium can be measured with ultrasound.

8.32 Lippes loop. Location of a Lippes loop inside the uterine cavity.

8.33 Two endometriotic (chocolate) cysts.

8.34 Polycystic ovaries. Ultrasound scanning of the pelvis provides the simplest method of diagnosing polycystic ovaries. Multiple small cysts can be seen throughout the ovarian cortex.

8.35 Multiple large ovarian cysts. Grossly hyperstimulated ovaries showing multiple large ovarian cysts.

8.36 A solitary, simple ovarian cyst.

8.37 A solitary, intramural uterine fibroid.

Magnetic resonance imaging

The use of magnetic resonance imaging (MRI) has been limited in obstetrics, but is more widespread in gynaecology (**8.38–8.44**). It depends on the use of powerful magnetic fields and pulsed radio frequencies to create maps of proton densities that give a high quality image of physical structure. With the use of spectroscopy, it can also be used to image biochemical reactions, but this has not been fully exploited in clinical imaging in obstetrics and gynaecology.

Fetus and placenta: magnetic resonance images

8.38 A normal fetus (sagittal view) at 36 weeks' gestation. This shows the fetal brain, the placenta, and fetal lung using a T2-weighted sequence.

8.39 A posterior, low-lying placenta. The internal cervical os can be clearly visualised, allowing precise placental localisation.

8.40 Umbilical cord at the abdominal insertion.

8.41 Buccal fat in a full term fetus. T1-weighted sequence highlighting the buccal fat in a full term fetus.

Gynaecology: magnetic resonance images

8.42 A normal pelvis. This demonstrates the harsh white appearance of the endometrium, the non-resonant subendometrial zone, and the clear outline of the myometrium.

8.43 Hydatidiform mole. Molar tissue can be seen invading the uterine wall.

8.44 Ovarian carcinoma. Different imaging sequences of an ovarian carcinoma. These highlight the interval structure of the tumour. Top left T_1/T_2;. top right STIR sequence; bottom left T_2;. bottom right T_1.

9. Gynaecology

Understanding the anatomy (**9.1–9.16**) and histology (**9.17–9.22**) of the pelvic organs is fundamental to understanding the range and effects of pelvic pathology. The relationship of the major organs within the pelvic cavity determines the course of malignant disease of the cervix and corpus uteri. Furthermore, understanding the processes involved in fertilisation and implantation depends on an appreciation of the cyclical changes in the endometrium and their relationship to the corresponding hormonal changes in the healthy sexually mature female.

The pathology of the pelvis and the female pelvic organs is extensive and varied. The ovary produces tumours of remarkable complexity and variability because it is totipotential. This atlas shows examples of the wide range of conditions, both congenital and acquired, encountered in the practice of gynaecology.

Anatomy of the pelvic organs

9.1 (left) Looking into the pelvis at the time of hysterectomy. The fundus of the uterus can be seen with the right fallopian tube emerging from the uterine fundus.

9.2 (right) Looking into the pelvis at the time of hysterectomy. The left tube and ovary can be seen lying on the posterior leaf of the broad ligament.

9.3 The uterus, tubes, and ovaries. Removed at the time of pelvic clearance.

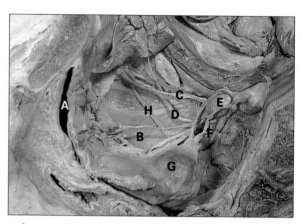

9.4 Gross hemisection of the pelvis. This shows the midline viscera and structures on the pelvic side wall. The dissection shows the obturator artery, vein, and nerve. In addition, the uterine artery and ureter, umbilical artery, ovary, and broad ligament can be seen.

9.5 Uterus, vagina and cervix. Close-up view of a dissection showing the cervix protruding into the vaginal vault.

A	Bladder	P	Ischiocavernosus
B	Ureter	Q	Bulbospongiosus
C	Obturator nerve	R	Small intestine
D	Obturator artery	S	Venous plexus
E	Ovary	T	Levator ani
F	Broad ligament	U	Ischial ramus
G	Uterus	V	Obturator internus
H	Obturator vein		
I	Vagina	W	Superior pubic ramus
J	Cervix		
K	Uterine tube	X	Pubis
L	Rectum	Y	Promontory of sacrum
M	Intestine		
N	Anal canal	Z	Cauda equina
O	Symphysis		

9.6 (left) Hemisection of the pelvis. This shows mid-line viscera, bladder, rectum, uterus, broad ligament, and ovary. Side wall left undissected, but external iliac vessels visible at pelvic brim.

9.7 (right) Sagittal section through the pelvis. This shows coils of gut, bladder, uterus, vagina, rectum, anal canal, ischiocavernosus, and bulbospongiosis muscles.

9.8 (left) The opposite side of 9.7. Gluteus maximus, a plexus of vessels around the vagina, levator ani muscle, obturator internus muscle, bladder, gut, and uterus can be identified.

9.9 (right) A parasagittal section. This shows similar features to **9.8**.

A	Small intestine
B	Sigmoid colon
C	Bladder
D	Gluteal muscles
E	Coils of small intestine
F	Trigone
G	Obturator internus
H	Obturator externus
I	Levator ani
J	Sacrum
K	Piriformis
L	Broad ligament
M	Uterus
N	Symphysis
O	Rectum
P	External iliac artery and vein
Q	Roof of acetabulum
R	Rectal ampulla
S	Femoral artery and vein
T	Obturator neurovascular bundle
U	Urethra
V	Vagina
W	Ischiorectal fossa
X	Anal canal
Y	Gluteus maximus
Z	Clitoris

9.10 Vertical section through the pelvis in a coronal plane. The hip joints and surrounding muscles can be seen, as well as the bladder, levator ani muscle, and coils of intestine.

9.11 Vertical section in a coronal plane. This shows the vagina as well as a profile of the bladder trigone with the ureteric orifices.

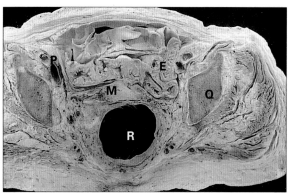

9.12 Horizontal section through the pelvis. This shows sacrum piriformis muscle, rectum, uterus, coils of gut, and gluteus maximus and medius muscles.

9.13 Section taken 2 cm below 9.13. This shows the rectal ampulla, uterus, ureter, coils of gut, external iliac vessels, and the coccyx.

9.14 Section taken 4 cm below 9.13. The rectal ampulla, vagina, and bladder can be seen, as well as the obturator internus muscle, gluteus maximus muscle, the inferior vessels, the ischiorectal fossa, and the hip joints.

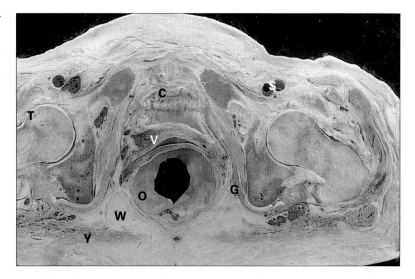

9.15 Section taken 2 cm below 9.14. This shows the anal canal, ischiorectal fossa, vagina, urethra, obturator internus muscle, levator ani muscle, and clitoris.

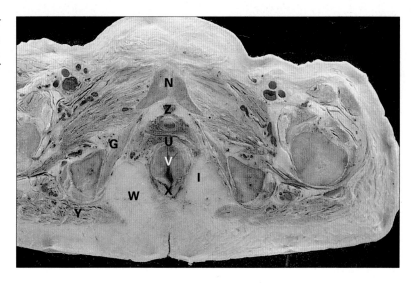

Histology of the endometrium

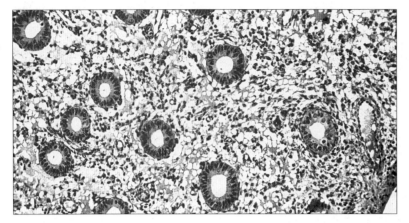

9.16 Proliferative phase of the endometrium. The surface epithelium is low and cuboidal. The glands are straight with no tendency to convolution. The stroma appears dense, compact, and non-vascular.

9.17 Early secretory phase endometrium. The surface epithelium is taller and definitely columnar and the glands become hypertrophic and convoluted, with evidence of secretory activity.

9.18 Mid-secretory phase. The secretory activity of the epithelium becomes increasingly marked, with glycogen granules in the epithelium and sometimes in the lumina of the glands.

9.19 Late secretory phase endometrium. This shows glandular as well as stromal changes. The saw-tooth pattern is characteristic and there is stromal invasion by 'pseudo-inflammatory cells'.

9.20 Menstrual endometrium. There is marked cellular infiltration of the upper layer, accompanied by small haematomas and surface tissue loss.

9.21 Decidualised endometrium. Stromal cells become large and polygonal with a wide zone of cytoplasm surrounding the nucleus. The decidual cells are arranged in a mosaic or tile-like fashion.

9.22 'Pill effect'. This shows the paucity of glandular activity and the decidual appearance of the stroma.

10. Lesions of the vulva and vagina

Examination of the vulva is an integral and important part of every gynaecological examination. The appearance of the vulva and vagina varies normally in relation to age and hormone status and changes in the skin of the vulva and vagina must take into account the expected texture of the epithelium for any given age. Good lighting and, where indicated, a magnifying glass or a colposcope, are needed for a systematic examination.

Both benign and malignant tumours of the vulva and vagina are relatively uncommon.

Congenital abnormalities of the vagina

The simplest vaginal abnormality which is easily treated by incision is the imperforate hymen (**10.1**). Congenital absence of the vagina results from defective formation of the müllerian ducts, and can be remedied by creating a space between the bladder and rectum, and inserting a mould covered by amnion or skin (**10.2–10.7**). The uterus is sometimes present, but has no external vaginal passage. Under these circumstances, a vagina must be created and the uterus connected to this cavity (**10.8–10.14**).

Congenital septum of the vagina can be easily divided, but is often asymptomatic (**10.15**).

10.1 Imperforate hymen. Menstrual loss has accumulated in the vagina and can be seen bulging the hymen.

10.2 Vaginal agenesis. The indentation over the normal site of the vaginal introitus can be seen. The uterus was absent in this patient, but the ovaries were present and the development of secondary sexual characteristics was normal.

10.3 Vaginal agenesis: surgery. Creation of a canal between the bladder and rectum allows the insertion of a mould in order to create an artificial vagina.

10.4 Vaginal agenesis: surgery. The remnants of the müllerian ducts may be demonstrated after reflection of the surface epithelium.

10.5 Vaginal agenesis: surgery. A space is created between the bladder and rectum.

10.6 Vaginal agenesis: surgery. It is important to achieve haemostasis if the amnion graft is to be retained.

10.7 Vaginal agenesis: surgery. An inflatable plastic mould is sutured into the vagina and held in place by labial closure. The mould can be reinflated by injecting fluid into the reservoir.

10.8 Vaginal agenesis. This woman presented with pain every month and was subsequently shown to have uterine tissue with a haematometra.

10.9 Vaginal agenesis. The uterus is distended and retrograde spill of menstrual loss had led to the development of endometriotic patches.

10.10 Vaginal agenesis. The uterine cavity is opened. It contains old, altered menstrual loss.

10.11 Vaginal agenesis: surgery. A catheter is inserted into the uterine cavity to connect it with the vaginal cavity.

10.12 Vaginal agenesis: surgery. Closure of the uterine incision after insertion of the uterine catheter.

10.13 Vaginal agenesis: surgery. An inflatable vaginal mould is inserted into the vaginal space.

10.14 Vaginal agenesis: surgery. Two catheters—one from the uterine cavity and one from the vaginal space—are shown draining the vulval wound.

10.15 Congenital septum of the vagina. This can be easily divided. The patient may present with dyspareunia or postcoital bleeding, but is often asymptomatic.

Lesions of the vulva

Various benign lesions of the vulva are demonstrated. These may be acquired or neoplastic (**10.16–10.21**), or congenital (**10.16**).

Vaginal prolapse is commonly, but not invariably, associated with uterine descent, and results in protrusion of both the anterior vaginal wall (cystocele) and posterior vaginal wall (rectocele) (**10.22–10.24**).Urethral caruncles are common (**10.25**), whereas clitoral hypertrophy (**10.26**) is relatively rare. **10.27** shows a gross example of herpetic vulvitis.

10.16 Vulval lipomas.

10.17 Benign vulval cyst. A large Wolffian duct cyst arising from a vestige of the Wolffian duct.

10.18 Benign vulval cyst: surgery. An incision is made through the labial skin to expose the cyst.

10.19 Benign vulval cyst: surgery. The cyst is fully exposed and dissected free from its underlying bed.

10.20 Benign   vulval   cyst: surgery. The wound is closed after excision of the cyst.

10.21 Large benign cystic tumour of the vulva.

10.22 Procidentia. A third-degree prolapse of the uterus and vaginal walls.

10.23 Procidentia with a large cystocoele.

10.24 Procidentia. Procidentia associated with dependent ulceration of the vaginal skin.

10.25 Urethral caruncle. The caruncle is a reddened, tender polypoid lesion arising from the posterior portion of the urethral meatus.

10.26 Clitoral enlargement associated with increased androgen secretion from an arrhenoblastoma.

10.27 Herpetic vulvitis. This infection is caused by herpes simplex virus. Lesions can occur in the cervix and in the perivulvar region.

Vulvar disease

The classification of vulvar disease depends on histological examination of a skin biopsy. Classification of vulval dystrophies is now listed as shown in Table 10.1.

Some examples of vulval dystrophies are shown (**10.28–10.32**). The majority of vulval carcinomas are squamous cell lesions, and are generally exophytic in nature (**10.33–10.35**).

Table 10.1 Classification of vulval dystrophies

I Non-neoplastic epithelial disorders of skin and mucosa
 1 Lichen sclerosus (lichen sclerosus et atrophicus)
 2 Squamous cell hyperplasia (formerly hyperplastic dystrophy)
 3 Other dermatoses

II Vulvar intra-epithelial neoplasia (VIN)
 VINI Mild dysplasia (formerly mild atypia)
 VINII Moderate dysplasia (formerly moderate atypia)
 VINIII Severe dysplasia (formerly severe atypia)
 VINIV Carcinoma *in situ*

10.28 Lichen sclerosus. Histological findings are thinning of the epidermis, subepidermal hyalinisation, and the presence of a deep band of inflammatory cells.

10.29 Leukoplakic vulvitis. Leukoplakic changes are associated with hyperkeratosis, irregular rete pegs, and dermal collagenisation.

10.30 Basal cell carcinoma of the vulva. This is involving the right labium majus.

10.31 Basal cell carcinoma of the vulva. Close-up view.

10.32 (left) Pigmented intraepithelial neoplasia or Bowen's disease of the vulva.

10.33 (right) Exophytic vulval carcinoma. The tumour is fungating and infected, with areas of necrosis.

10.34 Ulcerative squamous cell carcinoma of the vulva. Most of these tumours are squamous cell carcinomas.

10.35 Fungating squamous cell carcinoma of the vulva.

11. The cervix

The cervix uteri is the portion of the uterus that lies below the internal cervical os. It responds to the hormonal changes of the menstrual cycle. The changes are less obvious than those seen in the endometrium, but are particularly clear during the course of pregnancy.

The epithelium of the cervix is of two types. The section that protrudes into the vagina is lined by stratified squamous epithelium. The epithelium of the endocervix is lined by a cylindrical 'picket-fence' type of endocervical epithelium. This is much taller than the epithelium of the endometrium. The nuclei of the lining cells are placed basally. The glands of the cervix are of the racemose type and this epithelium normally shows no cornification. The transition may be sudden as the external epithelium joins the squamous epithelium at the squamocolumnar junction. The glands of the cervix are lined by epithelium similar to that which lines the endocervix.

The stroma of the cervix consists primarily of connective tissue with an increasing admixture of muscle cells as it nears the internal os. During pregnancy, there is a marked increase in the actual number of glands and the glands are increased in size and tortuosity, making up half the bulk of the cervix. There is also hyperplasia of the glandular epithelium.

Decidual reaction within a mosaic pattern in the stroma of the cervix suggests the presence of stromal cells within the stroma.

Examinations of the appearances of the normal cervix and of various pathological conditions are shown (**11.1–11.8**). Cervical cytology is an essential component of any cervical examination; (**11.19–11.22**) demonstrate the microscopic appearances of the cellular components of the smear..

11.1 Examination of the cervix. This can be achieved by direct inspection or by inspection through the colposcope.

11.2 Cervical cytology. This forms the basis of screening programmes for carcinoma of the cervix and is a routine part of the vaginal examination.

11.3 Normal multiparous cervix. The normal multiparous cervix treated with a dilute solution of acetic acid.

11.4 Normal cervix. Stained with Schiller's iodine. The squamocolumnar junction can be seen because only normal squamous epithelium stains.

11.5 (left) Fibroid polyp protruding through the external cervical os. This polyp probably arises within the uterine cavity.

11.6 (right) Small endocervical polyp. Such polyps may be lined with either squamous or columnar epithelium.

11.7 Cervical intraepithelial neoplasia (CIN) stage I. Acetowhite appearance of part of the anterior lip of the cervix associated with cervical intraepithelial neoplasia (CIN) Stage I. This relates to mild dyskaryosis in the cervical smear.

11.8 CIN2. The degree of histological abnormality is reflected in the intercapillary distance.

11.9 CIN2. The abnormal epithelium fails to stain with iodine.

11.10 CIN3. The lesion is predominantly around the external os.

11.11 CIN3. Histological examination of a biopsy taken from the non-staining area shows mitotic figures scattered throughout the thickness of the epithelium with no surface stratification.

11.12 CIN3. A further example. It is difficult to differentiate the grading of CIN by the colposcopic appearances.

11.13 CIN3. The non-iodine staining areas can be seen around the external os.

11.14 Human papilloma virus infection. Colposcopic appearances of human papilloma virus infection before the application of acetic acid.

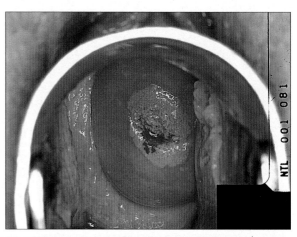

11.15 Human papilloma virus infection. A further example of human papilloma virus infection of the cervix.

11.16 Human papilloma virus infection. The same cervix stained with Lugol's iodine. The limits of the abnormal epithelium are clearly demarcated.

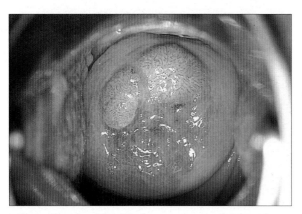

11.17 Cervical condylomata acuminata. These are gross lesions arising from tumour papilloma virus infection and are exophytic with multiple fine finger-like projections.

11.18 Exophytic invasive squamous cell carcinoma of the cervix.

Cervical cytology

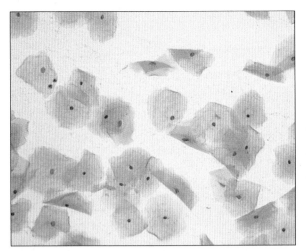

11.19 Normal cervical smear showing exfoliated cervical cells. Note the tiny nuclear remnants relative to the large volume of cytoplasm in each cell. (H & E stain; magnification x 65.)

11.20 Human papilloma virus. Numerous koilocytes can be seen. These cells show cytoplasmic vacuolation due to cytoplasmic necrosis. Occasionally, binucleate cells are also present.

11.21 Moderate dyskaryosis. Note that compared to the normal cells seen in **11.19** the abnormal cells are much smaller, but the nuclear/cytoplasmic ratio is approximately 50%. The nuclei vary in size and shape and chromatin distribution is irregular.

11.22 Carcinoma cells. Note the very large nuclei with marked abnormality of the chromatin distribution and the very large nuclear/cytoplasmic ratio. (Magnification x 65.)

12. Lesions of the uterus and fallopian tubes

Developmental abnormalities

The uterus forms as the result of fusion of the two müllerian ducts. This process gives rise to the upper two-thirds of the vagina, the cervix, and the body of the uterus. A range of abnormalities may arise as the result of malfusion or non-development of the müllerian ducts. The most common abnormalities of the uterus include the following:

- The presence of a septum (subseptate uterus).
- Non-fusion of the two uterine horns to form a bicornuate uterus with a single cervix (**12.1–12.5**).

12.1 Bicornuate uterus. One horn is enlarged by a fibroid and there is a single cervix. Uterus bicornis unicollis.

12.2 Bicornuate uterus. A further example of uterus bicornis unicollis.

12.3 Bicornuate uterus: surgery. Metroplasty for unification of a bicornuate uterus. A transverse incision is made across the uterine fundus to expose the cavity of the uterus and the midline septum. Note that externally the uterine fundus appears normal.

12.4 Bicornuate uterus: surgery. Once the septum is divided by diathermy, the uterine incision is closed anteroposteriorly.

12.5 Bicornuate uterus: surgery. When closure of the uterus is complete, the cavity is enlarged anteroposteriorly. This ensures that the two cut surfaces of the septum do not adhere together.

Tumours

Tumours involving the body of the uterus arise either from the endometrium or the myometrium and may be benign or malignant (**12.6–12.19**).

● The most common benign tumours of the endometrium are endometrial polyps.

● The most common tumours of the myometrium are uterine myomas. Fibroids occur in approximately 20 % of women over 30 years of age and in most women do not cause symptoms.

Approximately 67 % of women with carcinoma of the endometrium present after the menopause. The peak age incidence is 65.4 years.

Malignant tumours of the myometrium are very rare and have a particularly poor prognosis. Tumours of the fallopian tubes are exceedingly rare and account for no more than 0.2 % of all gynaecological malignancies.

12.6 Uterine fibroid. Lower abdominal distension arising from a large uterine fibroid. The patient had a palpable mass in her lower abdomen, but was otherwise asymptomatic.

12.7 Uterine fibroid. The grossly enlarged uterus is lifted out of the abdominal cavity at hysterectomy.

12.8 Uterine fibroid. The uterus is irregular because it contains multiple intramural fibroids.

12.9 Uterine fibroid. The size of the uterus in this case can be seen in the final specimen.

12.10 Multiple uterine fibroids. A further example of benign multiple uterine fibroids. This patient had severe menorrhagia.

12.11 Multiple uterine fibroids. The ovaries in this case were also enlarged with multiple small cysts and the tubes were engorged and highly vascular.

12.12 (left) Endometrial polyp. It is protruding through the cervical os.

12.13 (right) Submucous fibroid. This is contained within the cavity of the uterus and was causing menorrhagia and dysmenorrhoea.

12.14 (left) Fibroid polyp. This is protruding through the external cervical os, but arises from within the cavity of the uterus.

12.15 (right) Large degenerating fibroid. This shows evidence of calcification.

12.16 Large mixed Müllerian duct tumour. These tumours are rare, but are generally highly malignant variants of uterine sarcomas.

12.17 Large endometrial carcinoma. Multiple sections showing a large endometrial carcinoma invading the substance of the myometrium.

12.18 (left) Hydatidiform mole. This photograph of a hysterectomy specimen was taken in 1965. It is now very rare to resort to hysterotomy for evacuation of molar tissue because most trophoblastic tumours are now removed by suction evacuation. The molar tissue can be seen filling the cavity of the uterus.

12.19 (right) Hydatidiform mole. Dish containing the molar tissue after evacuation of the uterine cavity.

Endometriosis

Some aspects of endometriosis, particularly those deposits that arise outside the pelvic organs, are included in this chapter (**12.20–12.23**), while examples of ovarian endometriosis are included in Chapter 13.

12.20 Endometriosis in a Caesarean section scar. The dark, tender mass at the left extremity of the wound becomes particularly painful and enlarged during menstruation.

12.21 Umbilical endometriosis. This patient bled from her umbilicus during menstruation. Superficial diathermy of the lesion in her umbilicus did not help and later it was necessary to excise the umbilicus. Intense scarring can be seen in the subumbilical tissue.

12.22 Umbilical endometriosis. A low power view of the H & E section shows active endometrial deposits within the scar tissue.

12.23 Umbilical endometriosis. Higher powered magnification shows the active epithelial lining of the cavity of the endometriotic deposits.

Lesions of the fallopian tube

The most common cause of tubal disease is bacterial infection. Acute salpingitis may result from sexually transmitted infection and the acute condition may progress to a state of chronic salpingitis and tubal obstruction (**12.24–12.28**). Carcinoma of the fallopian tube (**12.29**) is an exceedingly rare tumour which produces a "canary yellow" vaginal discharge and is often diagnosed late. Severe pelvic inflammatory disease is another cause of tubal lesions (**12.26–12.28**).

Tubal patency can be demonstrated radiologically by the injection of a radio-opaque dye through the cervix (**12.30**).

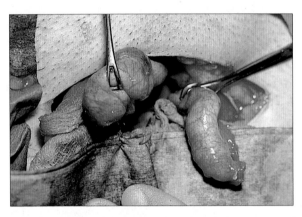

12.24 Acute salpingitis. This shows the engorged swollen tubes associated with acute infection. The pelvis is relatively free of adhesions at this stage.

12.25 Acute salpingitis. Beads of pus can be seen exuding from the fimbrial end of the tube.

12.26 Chronic pelvic inflammatory disease. Laparoscopic view of the pelvis in chronic pelvic inflammatory disease. The pelvis is partly obscured by adherent bowel and omentum.

12.27 Chronic pelvic inflammatory disease. Omentum adherent over the right tube, which is swollen and occluded. The fimbrial ends of the tube have disappeared and this is now a hydrosalpinx.

12.28 Chronic pelvic inflammatory disease. A sheet of fine adhesions cover the tubes and ovary, which is buried beneath the tube.

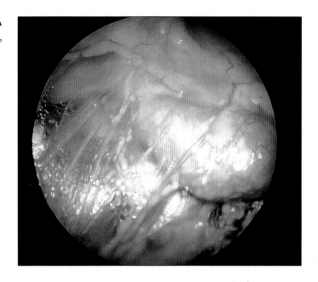

12.29 Carcinoma of the fallopian tube. This is a rare tumour with a highly malignant potential. It generally presents late.

12.30 Evaluation of tubal function. This is performed either by insufflation with dye or radiologically, as shown here, by the injection of radio-opaque dye. The triangular outline of the uterine cavity can be seen and the spill of dye on both sides from the fimbrial ends of the tubes. The dye spreads over the adjacent bowel.

13. Lesions of the ovary

The ovary is totipotential. Its structure varies on a cyclical basis and it produces the female sex hormones and the oocytes containing the genetic material of the mother. It is therefore not surprising that cystic and solid tumours of the ovary are common.

Ovarian lesions are commonly asymptomatic unless they undergo a complication such as torsion, rupture, haemorrhage, or necrosis. Signs of hormone-secreting tumours include virilisation or exaggerated female development, an abnormal menstrual cycle and precocious puberty.

Organic tumours of the ovary may be solid or cystic, benign or malignant. The ovary is also a common site of secondary tumours, particularly from primary sites in the breast and gastrointestinal tract.

Various examples of ovarian cysts, including those arising as a result of endometriosis, are demonstrated in **13.1–13.11**.

Follicular cyst

13.1 Single follicular cyst. Cross section of a normal ovary showing a single follicular cyst near the surface of the ovary and close to the ovarian hilus.

13.2 Small follicular cyst near mid-cycle. Surface appearance.

Endometriosis

13.3 Endometriotic patches on the surface of the ovary.

13.4 Bilateral ovarian enlargement. Both ovaries are affected by endometriosis and adherent behind the uterus.

13.5 Ruptured endometrioma. Chocolate fluid from a ruptured endometrioma of the ovary.

13.6 Endometrioma. Intact endometrioma of the ovary removed with the uterus at hysterectomy.

13.7 Bilateral ovarian endometriomas. Removed at hysterectomy.

13.8 Endometriomatous 'plaque' on the uterine fundus seen at the top side of this photograph with old altered blood on the adjoining surface.

13.9 Endometriosis. Bowel and omentum adherent to the left ovary by endometriosis, identified at laparoscopy.

13.10 Endometriosis. The same case as shown in **13.9**. An endometrioma can be seen on the left side in front of the ovary.

13.11 Endometriosis. The probe demonstrates adhesions to the tube and ovary to the posterior leaf of the broad ligament.

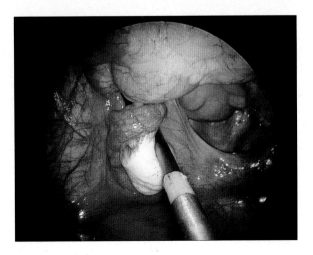

Benign cysts

Benign cysts of the ovary (**13.12–13.18**) are either functional or neoplastic.

● Functional cysts are rarely larger than 6 cm in diameter and are much more common than any other tumours of the ovaries. These cysts are follicular or lutein in origin and commonly occur in association with stimulation by gonadotrophins.

● Polycystic ovarian disease is associated with the presence of multiple small cysts in the ovary.

● Benign neoplastic tumours are epithelial in origin or arise from sex cord stroma or germ cell lines.

● Endometriotic cysts are common in the ovary.
 All these benign lesions have malignant variants.

13.12 Bilateral dermoid cysts demonstrated at laparotomy.

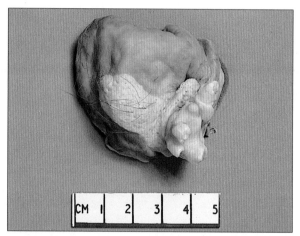

13.13 Dermoid cyst. Contents of a benign cystic teratoma or dermoid cyst showing teeth and hair.

13.14 Large benign ovarian serous cystadenoma at laparotomy.

13.15 Large benign ovarian serous cystadenoma. The tumour is delivered through the abdominal wound before removal.

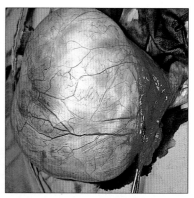

13.17 Large benign fimbrial cyst. The fine vascular structure of the cyst wall is reinforced after reflection of the tube.

13.18 Large benign fimbrial cyst. Removal of the intact fimbrial cyst.

13.16 Large benign fimbrial cyst. The tube can be seen spread over the cyst.

Malignant tumours of the ovary

The prognosis of malignant tumours of the ovary (**13.19–13.25**) is poor because spread is transcoelomic and occurs as soon as the surface of the ovary is breached by the tumour. Carcinoma of the ovary accounts for 5 % of all cancer deaths in women and the 5-year survival rate is only 25–30 %. This is because 75 % of such tumours present at an advanced stage.

Sex cord tumours are relatively rare (**13.26–13.31**) and are commonly hormone secreting. Androblastomas and Sertoli–Leydig cell tumours produce androgens and therefore exhibit signs of virilisation with increased facial hair, deepening of the voice and clitoral enlargement. On the other hand, granulosa cell tumours and thecomas produce oestrogen, and may cause precocious sexual development.

13.19 Ovarian adenocarcinomas. Removal of bilateral malignant ovarian adenocarcinomas.

13.20 Large endometrioid carcinoma of the ovary. The tumour is part cystic, part solid. The contralateral ovary is unaffected.

13.21 Large malignant ovarian tumour. Massive abdominal distension by a large malignant ovarian tumour.

13.22 Advanced mucinous cystadenocarcinoma of the ovary. Extensive omental tumour infiltrating from an advanced mucinous cystadenocarcinoma of the ovary.

13.23 Advanced mucinous cystadenocarcinoma of the ovary. Exposure of the tumour mass.

13.24 Advanced mucinous cystadenocarcinoma of the ovary. The final tumour specimen after excision.

13.25 Bilateral multicystic malignant ovarian tumours.

13.26 Androblastoma or Sertoli–Leydig cell tumour. Cross hemisection. These tumours produce testosterone and have relatively low malignant potential.

13.27 A Sertoli–Leydig cell tumour. About 50 % of these tumours produce androgen and virilisation.

13.28 Granulosa/theca cell tumour. This shows haemorrhagic areas in the solid white cut surface of the tumour. These tumours have low malignant potential, with reported 5-year survival rates at 60–90 %.

13.29 A large thecoma or theca cell tumour. The cut surface is yellow, reflecting the presence of neutral lipid.

13.30 Thecoma. Although thecomas are generally benign, if they secrete oestrogens they may cause, as in this case, an endometrial carcinoma. The thecoma can be clearly seen in the right ovary.

13.31 Dysgerminoma of the ovary. These tumours have a solid, fleshy surface with a smooth lobulated exterior. The histological appearance is identical to that of a seminoma of the testis. The tumour is malignant, with a 5-year survival rate of 63 % when it has extended beyond the ovary.

14. Common gynaecological operations

It is important that those medical advisers who have a responsibility for counselling women with gynaecological disorders have some idea of what is involved in the commonly performed operations. This atlas has not been compiled as an atlas of gynaecological procedures, but nevertheless, we feel that it is essential to include some pictures of the most commonly performed gynaecological operations. We therefore include descriptions of abdominal (**14.1–14.16**) and vaginal hysterectomy (**14.17–14.34**), dilatation and curretage (**14.35–14.41**), diagnostic laparoscopy (**14.42–14.54**), open clip sterilisation (**14.55–14.57**), minimal invasive surgery (**14..58–14.66**) and laparoscopic oophorectomy (**14.67–14.71**).

Abdominal hysterectomy

14.1 Exposure of the right round ligament and broad ligament. The right side is anterior.

14.2 Placement of straight Kocher's forcep. Straight Kocher's forcep is placed across the Fallopian tube to the left, the round ligament to the right, and part of the broad ligament.

14.3 Division of the round ligament, isolation of the infundibulopelvic fold, division of the broad ligament. The round ligament is divided and the infundibulopelvic fold containing the ovarian vessels is isolated by pushing a finger through the broad ligament, which is then divided.

14.4 The ovarian and round ligaments are transfixed and sutured.

14.5 Isolation of the lateral aspects of the uterine fundus.

14.6 Dissection of the uterovesical fold. The uterovesical fold of peritoneum is dissected free from the uterus and cervix.

14.7 Division of the uterovesical fold. The uterovesical fold is divided with scissors on both sides of the uterus.

14.8 Exposure of the uterine vessels. The uterine vessels are now exposed at the junction of the cervix and the body of the uterus.

14.9 Clamps are now applied across the uterine vessels.

14.10 The clamps occlude all of the uterine vessels to the lateral margin of the uterus.

14.11 Division of the cardinal ligaments, opening of the vaginal vault. The cardinal ligaments are divided and the vaginal vault is opened to expose the cervix.

14.12 After removal of the uterus. The uterus has now been removed and the pedicles and vaginal vault are sutured. Haemostasis is secured.

14.13 After removal of the uterus. The rectum can be seen on the left and the sutures holding the round ligaments on the right.

14.14 Closure of the pelvic peritoneum. The pelvic peritoneum is closed with a peritoneal suture.

14.15 The operation is now complete.

14.16 The specimen consists of the uterus, tubes, and ovaries.

Vaginal hysterectomy

14.17 Preparation of the patient. The patient is placed in the lithotomy position, cleaned, draped and catheterised.

14.18 The cervix is grasped with a vulsellum. The cervix is visible at the introitus and there is a visible cystocoele.

14.19 Infiltration of the paracervical tissue. The paracervical tissue is infiltrated with saline with or without a vasoconstrictor.

14.20 Freeing the bladder. A triangle of anterior vaginal wall is excised over the cystocoele and the bladder is dissected free.

14.21 Demonstration of the enterocoele. The cervix is circumcised. The enterocoele is posterior to the cervix.

14.22 Incision of the peritoneum. The peritoneum of the uterovesical fold is incised with scissors.

14.23 Insertion of a pedicle needle under the left cardinal ligament. The lateral cervical ligaments are exposed and a pedicle needle is inserted under the left cardinal ligament.

14.24 Separation of the cardinal ligament from the cervix. The cardinal ligament is cut until it is separated from the lateral aspect of the cervix.

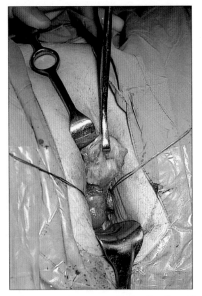

14.25 Exposure of the body of the uterus. The posterior peritoneum of the Pouch of Douglas is incised and the body of the uterus exposed.

14.26 The uterine vessels are clamped, cut, and transfixed.

14.27 Descent of the uterine body. The uterine body, which contains several small fibroids, now descends.

14.28 Cutting the pedicle. A clamp is applied across the round ligament, broad ligament, and Fallopian tube, and the pedicle is cut.

14.29 The uterine body and cervix are now delivered from the vagina.

14.30 Suturing the pedicles. The pedicles at the uterine horns are now sutured. The large bowel can be seen protruding through the peritoneal opening.

14.31 Closure of pelvic peritoneum. The pelvic peritoneum is now closed by cerclage, with exteriorisation of the pedicles.

14.32 The pedicles are tied together at the vaginal vault.

14.33 The pedicles are tied to the vaginal vault.

14.34 Closure of the anterior vaginal wall. This is completed with interrupted sutures.

Dilatation of the cervix and endometrial curettage

14.35 Preparation of the patient. The patient is placed in the lithotomy position, cleaned, draped, and catheterised.

14.36 Preoperative observation. The position, size, shape, and mobility of the uterus are noted before the procedure is commenced.

14.37 Exposure of the cervical os. A tenaculum is applied to the anterior lip of the cervix, a speculum is inserted, and the cervical os is clearly exposed.

14.38 Assessment of the uterus. The length and direction of the uterine cavity is measured and assessed with a sound.

14.39 Dilatation of the cervix. The cervix is dilated by introducing progressively larger cervical dilators.

14.40 Removal of any polyps. Polyp forceps are introduced into the uterine cavity, opened, rotated, closed, and withdrawn to attempt to grasp and remove any polyps.

14.41 Scrape of the uterine walls. A sharp uterine curette is inserted and the uterine walls are systematically scraped.

Laparascopy

14.42 Preparation of the patient. The patient is draped and the bladder is catheterised.

14.43 Vaginal examination is performed to determine the size and position of the uterus and whether there are any palpable adrenal masses.

14.44 Insertion of a Spackman's cannula. The cervix is grasped with a tenaculum and a Spackman's cannula is inserted to manipulate the uterus.

14.45 Insertion of a Spackman's cannula. The cannula is inserted to obtain a seal against the cervix.

14.46 Making a small subumbilical incision. A small subumbilical incision is made before insertion of the Verres needle for insufflation of gas into the peritoneal cavity.

14.47 Checking that the Verres needle is patent. The Verres needle is checked by gas insufflation to ensure that it is patent.

14.48 Insertion of the Verres needle. The needle is inserted into the abdominal cavity and care is taken to ensure that it has not been inserted into the bowel or major blood vessels. The abdomen is then distended with 3–4 litres of carbon dioxide or nitrous oxide.

14.49 Insertion of the trocar. The trocar is inserted downwards towards the pelvic cavity.

14.50 Visualisation of the pelvic organs. The uterus can now be manipulated to visualise the pelvic organs.

14.51 Insertion of a telescope. A telescope is inserted through the trocar and gas flow is sustained.

14.52 Making a small suprapubic incision. A small suprapubic incision is made for introducing a probe to manipulate and display the pelvic organs.

14.53 Insertion of the suprapubic Steptoe probe.

14.54 Expelling the gas and suturing the wound. On completion of the procedure, the gas is expelled and the subumbilical wound is sutured.

Open clip sterilisation

14.55 Application of a Filshie clip. The right fallopian tube is grasped with the clip.

14.56 The clip is closed and the tube is crushed.

14.57 Filshie clip in situ. The Filshie clip is closed and locked across the fallopian tube.

Minimal invasive surgery

The advent of suitable instrumentation has led to the development of minimal invasive surgery, with many new techniques designed to gain access to the pelvic organs with small abdominal incisions. Two of the procedures—endometrial resection and ablation (**14.58–14.63**) and laparoscopic oophorectomy (**14.64–14.68**)—are described here as examples of these innovations.

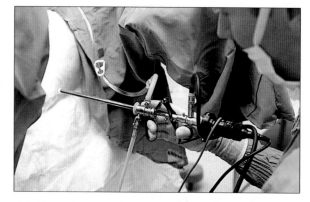

14.58 Endometrial resection and ablation. The patient is placed in the lithotomy position, cleansed, and draped, and the operating hysteroscope is introduced through the cervix.

14.59 Endometrial resection. After dilatation of the cervix, the resectoscope is inserted and the uterine cavity is distended with fluid. The endometrium is displayed on a television screen and the endometrium is resected.

14.60 Endometrial resection and ablation. 'Roller ball', used for diathermy, is placed inside the uterine cavity.

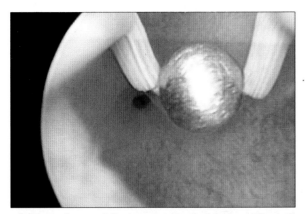

14.61 Endometrial resection and ablation. The ball is applied to the endometrium at the uterine fundus.

14.62 Endometrial resection and ablation. Diathermy of the endometrium in this fashion avoids preparation of the uterine fundus.

14.63 Endometrial resection and ablation. Endometrial resection is performed elsewhere in the uterine cavity with loop excision of the endometrium and underlying myometrium.

14.64 Endometrial resection and ablation. Furrow created by loop excision.

14.65 Endometrial resection and ablation. End result of endometrial resection.

14.66 Endometrial resection. Strips of endometrium and underlying myometrium are resected and removed through the cervix.

Laparoscopic oophorectomy

14.67 Laparoscopic oophorectomy. End of a large 10 mm grasper protruding through the cannula adjacent to the ovary.

14.68 Laparoscopic oophorectomy. Grasper is applied to the ovarian pedicle.

14.69 Laparoscopic oophorectomy. Filshie clip is used as a haemostat and applied across the ovarian pedicle.

14.70 Laparoscopic oophorectomy. Preparation of the pedicle for transsection after application of the Filshie clip.

14.71 Laparoscopic oophorectomy. Pedicle divided with removal of the ovary.

INDEX

abdomen, examination, 11–12, 15
abdominal cavity
  fetal ascites, 61
  inflation, 114
abdominal wall defect, 26, 61
abortion, missed, 62
acid-base balance, fetal, 31, 34
adnexal tumours, 15
adrenal hyperplasia, congenital, 28
alpha fetoprotein test, 23
amniocentesis, 23, 24
  needle, 24, 60
  ultrasound imaging, 60
amnion, 19, 20
  graft, 76
amnioscope, 34
amniotic fluid, 45
  aspiration, 24
  excess, 12
  fetal urine, 19
amniotic sac, 45
anaesthesia, regional, 49
anal canal, 69, 71
androblastoma, 103
androgen, 79, 103
anencephaly, 25, 60
antepartum monitoring, 31–4
aorta, fetal, 59
areola, 10
arrhenoblastoma, 79
ascites, fetal, 61
asphyxia, fetal, 31
Ayre's speculum, 16

basal nuclei, 61
bicornuate uterus, surgery, 89
biparietal diameter, 58
bladder, 68, 69, 70
  vaginal hysterectomy, 109
blastocoelic cavity, 18
blastocyst, 18
blood
  Doppler velocity measurement, 59
  fetal sampling, 59

  pressure, 9
bowel, fetal, 61
Bowen's disease of the vulva, 81
bradycardia, 33
brain, fetal
  cerebral ventricles, 59
  holoprosencephaly, 61
  magnetic resonance imaging (MRI), 64
breasts
  changes in pregnancy, 10
  gynaecological examination, 14
  lumps, 14
  striae gravidarum, 11
breech delivery, 37–41
  fetal descent, 38
  forceps, 37, 40
  sacral rotation, 39
broad ligament, 68, 69, 105, 110
buccal fat, fetal, 64
bulbospongiosus muscles, 69

Caesarean section, 43–9
  closure, 47–8
  delivery, 45–6
  endometriosis in scar, 93
  epidural anaesthesia, 49
  forceps, 46
  incidence, 43
  incision, 43–5
  placental delivery, 47
  postoperative complications, 43
  presenting part, 46
  upper segment, 43
carbon dioxide, 114
cardinal ligament, 107, 109
cardiotocography (CTG), 31, 32
cartilage development, 27
caudal regimen syndrome, 28
cephalopelvic disproportion, 43
cerebral ventricles, 59, 61
cervical cells, exfoliated, 87
cervical cytology, 83, 87
cervical dilators, 112
cervical intraepithelial neoplasia

stage 1 (CIN1), 84
stage 2 (CIN2), 84–5
stage 3 (CIN3), 85
cervical os, 64, 83, 84, 91, 112
cervical smear, 15, 16
  chromatin distribution, 87
  dyskaryosis, 84
  normal, 87
  nuclear/cytoplasmic ratio, 87
cervix, 83–7
  anatomy, 68
  carcinoma, 83, 86
  carcinoma cells, 87
  cardinal ligament separation, 109
  colposcopy, 16, 85, 86
  condylomata acuminata, 86
  cytoplasmic vacuolation, 87
  dilatation, 112
  dyskaryosis, 87
  epithelium, 16, 83
  examination, 15, 16, 83
  glands, 83
  herpetic lesions, 79
  human papilloma virus infection, 86
  malignant disease, 67
  necrosis, 87
  normal, 84
  paracervical tissue, 109
  pregnancy, 13
  removal, 110
  squamocolumnar junction, 83, 84
  squamous cell carcinoma, 86
  stroma, 83
  vaginal hysterectomy, 108
chloasma, 9
chocolate cysts, 63
chorion
  frondosum, 19
  laeve, 19
  villus sampling, 23
chorionic plate, 19
chromosome analysis 45XO, 28
cleavage, 18
cleft palate, 23
clitoris, 71, 78, 79
clitoromegaly, 28
coccyx, 13, 71
colostrum, 10
colposcope, 75, 83

colposcopic examination, 16, 83, 85, 86
condylomata acuminata, cervical, 86
congenital abnormalities, 23, 60–1
Copeland electrode, 32
cord traction, 35, 36, 41, 53
corpus uteri, 67
cotyledons, 20, 21
cranial vault, 61
crown–rump length, 19, 55
Cusco's speculum, 15
cystadenocarinoma, ovarian mucinous, 102
cystadenoma, benign ovarian serous, 100
cystic hygroma, 27
cystocoele, 78, 108, 109
  with procidentia, 79

delivery
  Caesarean section, 45–6
  low forceps, 50–3
  see also vaginal delivery, spontaneous
dermoid cysts, ovarian, 100
diabetes, maternal, 28, 29
diastolic blood pressure, 9
digestive enzymes, fetal, 19
Doppler blood velocity measurement, 59
Down's syndrome, 23, 28
dysgerminoma of ovary, 103
dysmenorrhoea, 91
dyspareunia, 77

egg
  one-cell, 17
  unfertilised, 17
embryo, six-cell, 18
encephalocoele, 27
endocervix, 83
endometrial carcinoma, ovarian, 103
endometrial resection and ablation, 116
endometrioma, ovarian, 98, 99
endometriosis, 76, 93
  adhesions, 99
  ovary, 98–9
  umbilical, 93
endometriotic cysts, 63
  ovarian, 100
endometrium
  benign tumours, 90

carcinoma, 90, 92
cyclical changes, 67
decidualised, 73
diathermy, 117
histology, 72–4
loop excision, 117
magnetic resonance imaging (MRI), 65
menstrual, 73
pill effect, 74
polyps, 90, 91
proliferative phase, 72
secretory phase, 72–3
stroma, 73, 74
ultrasound imaging, 62
endoscopy, fetal, 25
enterocoele, 109
epidural anaesthesia, 49
episiotomy
 breech delivery, 37
 closure, 41–2
 low forceps delivery, 50, 53
 repair, 41–2, 53
examination methods, 9–16
 abdomen, 11–12, 15
 gynaecological, 14–16
 pelvis, 13
exomphalos, 26, 61
external iliac vessel, 69, 71
eyes, fetal, 19

face
 bruising with spontaneous vaginal delivery, 36
 oedema, 29
 ultrasound imaging of fetal, 56
fallopian tube, 67, 68
 adhesions, 95
 carcinoma, 95
 endometriosis adhesions, 99
 Filshie clip, 115–16
 function evaluation, 95
 lesions, 94–5
 salpingitis, 94
 tumours, 90
female development, exaggerated, 97
fertilisation, 17, 67
fetal acid–base balance, 31, 34
fetal ascites, 61
fetal asphyxia, 31

fetal distress, 43
fetal ECG, 31
fetal heart
 auscultation, 12
 ultrasound imaging, 57, 58
fetal heart beat, 19
 absent, 62
fetal heart rate, 31
 variability, 32, 33
fetal membranes, 19, 20
fetal organs
 eviscerated, 61
 ultrasound imaging, 57
fetoscopy, 25
fetus
 blood sampling, 34, 59
 buccal fat, 64
 development, 11, 18, 19
 electrode, 32, 33
 hydropic, 27
 lie, 12
 magnetic resonance imaging (MRI), 64
 palpation, 12
 position of back, 12
 presenting part, 12
 respiration, 19
 ultrasound imaging, 55–61
 see also growth, fetal
fibroid polyp, 84
fibroids
 degenerating, 91
 submucous, 91
 uterine, 63, 90, 91
Filshie clip, 115–16
 ovarian pedicle, 118
fimbrial cyst, ovarian, 101
fluid thrill, 12
follicular cyst, 97
forceps
 breech delivery, 37, 40
 Caesarean section delivery, 46
 low forceps delivery, 50–3
 polyp, 113
fornices, palpation, 16
fundal pressure, 35, 36

gastroschisis, 61
genitalia, external fetal, 57

germinal vesicle, 17
gestational age
    conceptus size, 62
    ultrasound assessment, 55, 58
glomerular function, 19
glucose, urine analysis, 13
gluteus maximus muscle, 69, 71
glycogen granules, 72
goitre, 30
growth, fetal, 11
    abdominal circumference, 59
    asymmetrical retardation, 59
    head circumference measurement, 58
gut, 69, 71
    mucosal glands, 19
gynaecological conditions, 62–3
gynaecological examination, 14–16, 75
gynaecological operations, 105–18
gynaecological pathology diagnosis, 55
gynaecology, 67–74
    magnetic resonance imaging (MRI), 65

haematoma, endometrial, 73
haematometra, 76
haemostatic clamps, 47
hare lip, 23
HCG test, 23
head, fetal
    breech delivery, 37, 40
    Caesarean section delivery, 46
    circumference measurement, 58
    crowning, 51
    vaginal delivery, 35
heart disease, congenital, 23
    see also fetal heart
height, 9
herpes gestationis, 30
herpes simplex virus, 79
herpetic vulvitis, 78, 79
holoprosencephaly, 61
hormonal changes, 67
hormone secreting tumours, 97
human papilloma virus
    cervical cytology, 87
    infection, 86
hydatiform mole, 62, 65, 92
hydramnios, 12
hydrocephalus, 60
hydropic fetus, 27

hydrosalpinx, 94
21–hydroxylase deficiency, 28
hymen, imperforate, 75
hyperplastic dystrophy see vulva, squamous cell
hyperplasia
hysterectomy, 67, 90
    abdominal, 105–8
    endometrioma, 98
    hydatiform mole, 92
    vaginal, 108–11

implantation, 18, 67
infundibulopelvic fold, 105
insemination, subzonal, 17
intertuberous diameter, 13
intestine, 70
intrapartum monitoring, 31–4
ischial spines, 13
ischiocavernosus, 69
ischiorectal fossa, 71

ketone bodies, 13
kidney, fetal, 19
Kocher's forceps, 105
koilocytes, 87
Korotkoff fourth sound, 9

labio-scrotal fusion, 28
labour
    first stage, 33
    second stage, 29, 35
    third stage, 36, 41
laparoscopic oophorectomy, 118
laparoscopy, 113–15
levator ani muscle, 41–2, 69, 70, 71
lichen sclerosus, 80
limb development, 19
lipoma, vulval, 78
Lippes loop, 63
liver, fetal, 61
low forceps delivery, 50–3
    crowning of head, 51
    delivery, 51–2
    descent, 50–1
    episiotomy, 50, 53
    placental delivery, 53

lungs, fetal, 19

magnetic resonance imaging (MRI), 64–5
    buccal fat, 64
    fetal brain, 64
    gynaecology, 65
    hydatiform mole, 65
    normal fetus, 64
    ovarian carcinoma, 65
    pelvis, 65
    umbilical cord, 64
medius muscle, 71
menopause, 90
menorrhagia, 91
menstrual cycle
    abnormal, 97
    endometriosis, 93
    hormonal changes, 83
menstrual loss, 75, 76, 77
mental retardation, severe, 23
micro-injection, 17
Montgomery's tubercles, 10
morula, 18
Müllerian duct, 75, 89
    tumour, 92
myelomeningocoele, 25, 26
myometrium, 65
    benign tumours, 90
    endometrial carcinoma, 92
    loop excision, 117
    malignant tumours, 90, 92
    uterine myoma, 90

neural tube defect, 23, 26
nipple, 10
nitrous oxide, 114

obturator internus muscle, 69, 71
obturator nerve, 68
obturator vessels, 68
oedema
    facial, 29
    lower limb, 28
oestriol, serum, 23
oestrogen secretion, 103
oligohydramnios, 27

oocyte/cumulus complex, 17
oocytes, 17
    polar bodies, 17
    production, 97
    pronucleate, 18
oophorectomy, laparoscopic, 118
operative delivery
    Caesarean section, 43–9
    indications, 43
    low forceps, 50–3
organogenesis, 19
organs, fetal, 57, 61
ovarian ligament, 106
ovary
    adenocarcinoma, 101
    adhesions, 95, 99
    anatomy, 68, 69
    androblastoma, 103
    benign neoplastic tumours, 100
    bilateral enlargement, 98
    carcinoma, 65, 101
    cystic teratoma, 100
    cysts, 63, 91, 100–1
    dermoid cysts, 100
    dysgerminoma, 103
    endometrial carcinoma, 103
    endometriosis, 98–9
    endometriotic cysts, 100
    endometroid carcinoma, 101
    fimbrial cyst, 101
    follicular cyst, 97
    granulosa/theca cell tumour, 103
    hormone secreting tumours, 97
    lesions, 97–103
    malignant tumours, 101–4
    mucinous cystadenocarcinoma, 102
    multicystic malignant tumours, 102
    pedicle, 118
    polycystic, 63
    secondary tumours, 97
    serous cystadenoma, 100
    thecoma, 103
ovulation, 18

Pawlik's grip, 12
pedicle
    cutting, 110
    needle, 109

suturing, 110
    tying at vaginal vault, 111
pelvic cavity, 13
pelvic clearance, 68
pelvic examination, 13, 16
    speculum, 13, 15
pelvic inflammatory disease, chronic, 94, 95
pelvic inlet, 13
pelvic organs
    anatomy, 67–71
    bimanual palpation, 16
    histology, 72–4
    pathology, 67
    visualisation, 114
pelvic outlet, 13
pelvic peritoneum closure, 107, 111
pelvis
    anatomy, 67
    bony, 13
    funnel, 13
    hemisection, 68, 69
    horizontal section, 71
    magnetic resonance imaging (MRI), 65
    pathology, 67
    sagittal section, 69
    vertical section, 70
perineum, 50, 51
perivitelline space, 17
perivulvular region, 79
physical examination, 9
piezo–electric crystal, 55
pigmentation
    areolar, 10
    facial, 9
Pinard stethoscope, 12
piriformis muscle, 71
placenta
    Caesarean section delivery, 47
    circumvallate, 20
    delivery, 35, 36
    fetal surface, 19
    function, 19
    low forceps delivery, 53
    magnetic resonance imaging (MRI), 64
    maternal surface, 20
    posterior low-lying, 64
    praevia, 43
    retained tissue in uterus, 62

twin, 21
placental abruption, 21
polycystic ovarian disease, 100
polyp
    endocervical, 84
    endometrial, 90, 91
    fibroid, 84, 91
    forceps, 113
    uterine, 113
postcoital bleeding, 77
Potter's syndrome, 27
pouch of Douglas, 110
pre-eclampsia, 29, 43
precocious puberty, 97
pregnancy
    abnormalities, 55
    body changes, 9
    breasts, 10
    cervical stroma, 83
    cervix, 13
    mask, 9
    medical disorders, 29–30
    twin, 60
    ultrasound imaging, 55–61
    uterus, 13
    vaginal walls, 13
prenatal screening, 23
procidentia, 79
protein, urine analysis, 13
pseudo-inflammatory cells, 73

rectal ampulla, 71
rectocele, 78
rectum, 68, 69, 71
rectus sheath, 43–4, 48
renal agenesis, 27
renal tubules, 19
resectoscope, 116
respiration, fetal, 19
retained products of conception, 62
roller ball, 116
round ligament, 105, 106, 107, 110

sacral agenesis, 28
sacral curve, 13
sacral promontary, 13

salpingitis, 94
scalp, fetal
    blood sampling, 34
    electrode, 33
Sertoli–Leydig cell tumour, 103
sex, fetal, 19, 57
sex hormone production, 97
skin pigmentation, 9
small intestine, fetal, 61
Spackman's cannula, 113, 114
speculum, 13, 15
spermatozoa, 17
spina bifida, 57, 60
spine, fetal, 57
stem villus, 19
Steptoe probe, suprapubic, 115
striae gravidarum, 11
stromal cells, 83
subconjunctival ecchymosis, 29
subendometrial zone, 65
subpubic arch angle, 13
subumbilical incision, 114
suprapubic incision, 115
surgery, minimal invasive, 116
survival rate, ovarian malignant tumours, 101, 103
sutures, 41
    Caesarean section closure, 48
    episiotomy, 53

tachycardia, resting, 32
tenaculum, 112, 113
teratoma, benign cystic, 100
testosterone, 103
thecoma, 103
thyroid enlargement, 30
trisomy, 27
trocar, 114
    telescope insertion, 115
Turner's syndrome, 28
twin
    placenta, 21
    pregnancy, 60

ultrasound
    pulsed Doppler, 31
    screening, 23, 24
ultrasound imaging, 55–63

amniocentesis, 60
anencephaly, 60
cerebral ventricles, 59
congenital abnormalities, 60–1
endometriotic cysts, 63
endometrium, 62
exomphalos, 61
fetal aorta, 59
fetal ascites, 61
fetal bowel, 61
fetal heart, 57, 58
fetal organs, 57
fetal spine, 57
gestational age, 55, 58
gynaecological conditions, 62–3
holoprosencephaly, 61
hydatiform mole, 62
hydrocephalus, 60
image quality, 55
linear array scanners, 55
Lippes loop, 63
mechanical array scanners, 55
missed abortion, 62
ovarian cysts, 63
phased array scanners, 55
polycystic ovaries, 63
real time scanners, 55
retained products of conception, 62
spina bifida, 60
twin pregnancy, 60
umbilical cord, 59
uterine fibroid, 63
umbilical cord, 20
    blood sampling, 59
    clamping/cutting, 36, 47, 52
    low forceps delivery, 52
    magnetic resonance imaging (MRI), 64
    ultrasound imaging, 59
umbilical vessels, 20, 68
umbilicus, endometriosis, 93
ureter, 68, 71
ureteric orifices, 70
urethra, 71
    caruncle, 78, 79
urinalysis, 13
urine, fetal, 19
uterine activity recording, 31, 33
uterine body, 110
uterine cavity, 116

uterine contraction recording, 33
uterine curette, 113
uterine fundus, 11, 36, 106
uterine scar rupture risk, 43
uterine vessels, 68, 106–7, 110
uterine wall
   hydatiform mole, 65
   scraping, 113
uterovesical fold, 106, 109
uterus
   anatomy, 68, 69, 71
   bicornuate, 89
   developmental abnormalities, 89
   exposure of body, 110
   fibroid polyp, 91
   fibroids, 63, 90, 91
   fundus, 67
   incision, 45, 47
   lesions, 89–93
   Lippes loop, 63
   myoma, 90
   placental tissue retention, 62
   polyps, 113
   position, 13, 15
   pregnancy, 13
   prolapse, 79
   removal, 107
   sarcoma, 92
   shape, 15
   size, 13, 15
   subseptate, 89
   tumours, 90–2
   vaginal agenesis, 75, 76, 77

vagina
   amnion graft, 75, 76
   anatomy, 68, 69, 70, 71
   artificial, 75, 76, 77
   cervical cytology, 83
   congenital abnormalities, 75–7
   congenital septum, 75, 77
   examination, 15, 75, 83, 113
   laparoscopy, 113
   muscle plexus, 69
   prolapse, 78
   ulceration, 79
vaginal agenesis, 75–7

vaginal delivery, spontaneous, 35–6
   external rotation, 35
   face presentation, 36
   head, 35
   shoulders, 35
vaginal mould, inflatable, 75, 76, 77
vaginal vault, 107, 111
vaginal wall
   examination, 15
   posterior, 78
   pregnancy, 13
   prolapse, 79
   suture, 41
Verres needle, 114
villi, fetal, 20
virilisation, 97, 103
visceromegaly, 29
vulsellum, 108
vulva
   basal cell carcinoma, 80, 81
   benign cystic tumour, 78
   cyst, 78
   dystrophies, 80
   examination, 15, 75
   intra–epithelial neoplasia, 80, 81
   lesions, 78
   lipoma, 78
   squamous cell carcinoma, 81
   squamous cell hyperplasia, 80
vulvar disease, 80–1
vulvitis, leukoplakic, 80

weight, 9
Wharton's jelly, 20

zona pellucida, 17